COMPETENCIES
FOR THE PALLIATIVE AND HOSPICE
ADVANCED PRACTICE
REGISTERED NURSE

Third Edition

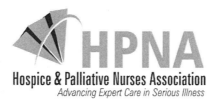

Constance Dahlin, MSN, ANP-BC, ACHPN, FPCN, FAAN
Consultant
Hospice and Palliative Nurses Association
Pittsburgh, PA

CONTRIBUTORS

Sarah F. D'Ambruoso, MSN, ACAGNP, ACHPN
Palliative Care Nurse Practitioner
UCLA Health
Santa Monica, CA

Anessa M. Foxwell, MSN, AGPCNP-BC, AGACNP-BC, ACHPN
Pre-doctoral Fellow, New Courtland Center for Transitions & Health University
of Pennsylvania School of Nursing
Nurse Practitioner
Penn Medicine
Philadelphia, PA

Marianne Johnstone-Petty, DNP, FNP-C, APRN, ACHPN
Director of Interprofessional Palliative Education
Palliative Care Department
Providence Medical Group
Anchorage, AK

Maura Farrell Miller, PhD, GNP-BC, APRN, PMHCNS-BC, ACHPN
Director
Hospice and Palliative Care Program
Department of Veterans Affairs Medical Center
West Palm Beach, FL

Barbara Reville, DNP, ANP-BC, ACHPN
Nursing Director, Adult Palliative Care
Department of Psychosocial Oncology and Palliative Care
Dana-Farber Cancer Institute
Fellowship Director, Palliative Care Nurse Practitioner Fellowship
Harvard Medical School Center for Palliative Care
Boston, MA

Lisa A. Stephens, MSN, ANP-BC, APRN, ACHPN, FPCN
Lead Nurse Practitioner
Associate Program Director, Hospice and Palliative Interprofessional Fellowship
Section of Palliative Medicine
Dartmouth-Hitchcock Medical Center
Lebanon, NH

Christine G. Westphal, MSN, NP, ACNS, ACHPN, FPCN
Palliative Care Nurse Practitioner
Beaumont Health
Dearborn, MI

Clareen Wiencek, PhD, ACNP-BC, CNP, ACHPN, FAAN
Professor of Nursing
Advanced Practice Program Director for MSN and DNP Programs
University of Virginia School of Nursing
Charlottesville, VA

Dorothy Wholihan, DNP, AGPCNP-BC, ACHPN, FPCN, FAAN
Clinical Professor
Director, Palliative Care Specialty Program
NYU Meyers College of Nursing
New York, NY

REVIEWERS

Carrie L. Cormack, DNP, CPNP, APRN, CHPPN
Assistant Professor
Pediatric Nurse Practitioner/Palliative Care
College of Nursing, Medical University of South Carolina
Charleston, SC

Nicole DePace, MS, GNP-BC, APRN, ACHPN
Director Palliative Care Consult Services
Palliative Nurse Practitioner
NVNA and Hospice
Norwell, MA

Jeanna Ford, DNP, ACNS-BC, APRN, ACHPN
Hematology-Oncology APC
Presbyterian Healthcare System
Albuquerque, NM

Jennifer Gentry, DNP, ANP-BC, GNP, ACHPN, FPCN
Nurse Practitioner
Palliative Care Consult Service
Duke University Hospital
Clinical Associate
Duke University School of Nursing
Durham, NC

Marika Haranis, MSN, FNP-BC, AGACNP-BC, ACHPN
System Clinical Director
Palliative Medicine and Comprehensive Care
Inova Health System
Falls Church, VA

Marianne Johnstone-Petty, DNP, FNP-C, APRN, ACHPN
Director of Interprofessional Palliative Education
Palliative Care Department
Providence Medical Group
Anchorage, AK

Maureen Lynch, MS, ANP-BC, ACHPN
Consultant
Millbury, MA

Lolita Melhado, PhD, FNP-BC, APRN, ACHPN
Assistant Professor
Doctor of Nursing Practice (DNP) Program Director
Florida Gulf Coast University School of Nursing
Vice President, Clinical Programs
One Accord Health
Fort Myers, FL

Lori S. Ruder, DNP, AGACNP-BC, APRN-CNP, ACHPN
Nurse Practitioner
Department of Palliative and Supportive Care
Cleveland Clinic Foundation
Cleveland, OH

Cheryl A. Thaxton, DNP, CPNP, FNP-BC, APRN, CHPPN, ACHPN, FPCN
Associate Clinical Professor
DNP Program Director/APRN Clinical Tracks
College of Nursing
Texas Woman's University
Dallas, TX

Phyllis Whitehead, PhD, CNS, APRN, ACHPN, RN-BC, FNAP
Clinical Ethicist
Clinical Nurse Specialist Palliative Medicine/Pain Management
Carilion Roanoke Memorial Hospital
Associate Professor
Virginia Tech Carilion School of Medicine
Roanoke, VA

Dorothy Wholihan, DNP, AGPCNP-BC, ACHPN, FPCN, FAAN
Clinical Professor
Director, Palliative Care Specialty Program
NYU Meyers College of Nursing
New York, NY

Alexander Wolf, DNP, ACNPC-AG, ACCNS-AG, ACHPN
Nurse Practitioner, Palliative Care
University of Cincinnati
Cincinnati, OH

Contents

Foreword

Overview of Palliative Nursing, Standards of Practice, and Competencies

Palliative nursing is recognized as a nursing specialty that encompasses a specified area of discrete study, research, and practice as defined and recognized by the profession.[1] Palliative nursing is the care delivered to individuals with serious illness, through the life cycle, regardless of prognosis. Individuals include perinates, neonates, infants, children, adolescents, young adults, and older adults. Hospice nursing is a subspecialty of palliative nursing and focuses on the specialized care of individuals with a terminal illness who have a prognosis of six months and want to focus on comfort care. Palliative care begins at diagnosis through end of life in many health settings: inpatient, home, or residential hospice; acute care hospitals or palliative care units; long-term care facilities; rehabilitation facilities; homes or residences; office-based clinics, such as palliative care, primary care, or disease clinics; veterans' facilities; correctional facilities; homeless shelters; and mental health and psychiatric settings.[2]

The American Nurses Association (ANA) requires that recognized specialties, such as palliative nursing, have a unique scope and standards of practice that delineate the components of professional nursing essential for that specialty. Specifically, a scope and standards describe the nature of a nursing specialty in terms of the work of the professional nurse and the responsibility of the specialty within itself and to the public.[1]

Palliative nursing was first recognized in 1987 and has an distinguished history and recognized presence in healthcare, with clearly defined scope and standards of practice, and a substantial number of members who devote most of their professional time to the specialty.[1,2] Palliative Nursing: Scope and Standards of Practice defines the practice of palliative nursing—who benefits from palliative nursing, what palliative nursing does, where palliative nursing is delivered, when palliative nursing is delivered, how palliative nursing is delivered, and why palliative nursing is a specialty.[1,2]

ANA requires specialty practice scope and standards to be updated at regular intervals to reflect the changing dynamics resulting in new patterns of professional practice and a shifting environment.[1] Revisions should incorporate new science, unveiling of the depth of health disparities, and care in natural disasters and public health crises within the nursing profession and the public. In addition, specific conditions and clinical circumstances may also affect the application of the standards at a given time (e.g., the time during a natural disaster, epidemic, or pandemic). Palliative Nursing: Scope and Standards of Practice have been recently revised to correspond to the current, dynamic environment.[2]

To complement the Palliative Nursing: Scope and Standards of Practice, palliative nursing has clinical nursing competencies. Competencies are the actions that reflect the integration of knowledge, skills, experience, and attitudes required to meet the clinical needs of individuals with serious illness, their families, and the public. There are competencies for the registered nurse (RN) and the advanced practice registered nurse (APRN). When a scope and standards of practice is revised, it is imperative to update specialty competencies to ensure congruency of practice expectations.

This third edition of Competencies for the Palliative and Hospice Advanced Practice Registered Nurse has been revised to represent the roles (e.g., clinical, research, education, administration, case management, administration, policy), settings (e.g., residential, home, acute care, office, clinic, hospice, skilled nursing facilities, assisted living), and range of populations (i.e., perinates, neonates, infants, children, adolescents, young adults, and older adults) encompassed in the palliative advanced practice registered nurse roles. The foundation of the competencies was developed by advanced practice nursing faculty and reviewed by palliative and hospice APRNs representative of the richness in diversity of practice in terms of geography, demography, setting of practice, population of focus, and areas of expertise.

History of the Palliative Advanced Practice Registered Nurse

Over the past 30 years, the development of palliative advanced practice nursing has been remarkable. In the late 1990s, there were very few APRNs specializing in palliative nursing.[3] In 2002, recognizing the growing expansion of the advanced practice nursing role in palliative care, a summit of advanced practice nurses representing clinical practice, research, and academics was convened to discuss the role and its impact in healthcare. The result was the white paper, *Advanced Practice Nurses Role in Palliative Care— A Position Statement from American Nursing Leaders,* which served as the foundation for the Hospice and Palliative Nurses Association (HPNA) position statement on *Value of the Advanced Practice Registered Nurse in Palliative Care.*[4,5] A major theme describing the role of palliative APRNs in 2001 remains current today: palliative and hospice APRNS are a valuable resource in healthcare reform who can further palliative care and nursing, promote access to palliative care, and direct palliative research.[4] The white paper and the position statement provided the foundation for the development of competencies to delineate the knowledge, skills, and attitudes for specialty palliative advanced practice nursing practice.

As a pivotal and integrated member of the interdisciplinary palliative care team, palliative and hospice APRNs promote wider access to palliative care services, and are a solution to clinical care, especially with the shortage within the palliative specialty workforce.[6] Twenty years later, palliative and hospice APRNs administer and lead programs, direct research, educate nurses on palliative care, and promote safe, quality, high-level care. These developments necessitate the revision of the competencies in order to bring them into concordance with current practice and expectations.

Much has changed in advanced practice palliative nursing since the development of the first edition of competencies. In 2002, there were only a handful of hospice and palliative APRNs across the country. Many received graduate education in related specialties, such as oncology, acute care, and geriatrics.[3] Now, there are several specialty palliative nursing master's programs and curricula developed for clinical nurse specialists and nurse practitioners who complete education in one of six foci delineated by the *APRN Consensus Model* as well as palliative care. There are several thousand hospice and palliative APRNs who practice in a variety of settings (e.g., home, skilled facilities, assisted living, hospices, hospitals, clinics).[7]

In 2002, specialty palliative and hospice advanced practice registered nurse (APRN) certification was in development by the National Board for Certification of Hospice and Palliative Nursing in collaboration with the American Nurses Credentialing Center. Currently, there are more than 2,200 hospice and palliative APRNs certified by Hospice and Palliative Care Credentialing Center.[7]

In 2002, The National Consensus Project for Quality Palliative Care (NCP) *Clinical Practice Guidelines for Quality Palliative Care* was in development and there was no core curriculum for advanced practice nurses. As of this writing, the NCP *Clinical Practice Guidelines*, which defines high-quality palliative care, is in its 4th edition.[8] The *Core Curriculum for Hospice and Palliative Advanced Practice Registered Nurse* is in its third edition.[9]

Five pillars of excellence guide the work of the HPNA: education, competence, advocacy, leadership, research, and scholarship.[10] Each pillar has specific indications for advanced practice nursing along with an additional pillar of clinical practice, which is highlighted in the Table 1 below.[6]

Table 1. HPNA Pillars and the APRN Role[3,11]

Pillar	Represented by HPNA as	The APRN Role
Education/ Continuing Professional Development	The association that serves as the primary resource and voice for the state-of-the-art and science palliative nursing knowledge.	Disseminates education that reflects the state-of-art and science in both the provision of palliative nursing as well as the continual pursuit of lifelong learning in the field (e.g., national and regional conferences, webinars, e-learning, journals, textbooks).
Continuing Competence	The association that empowers and facilitates its nurse members to demonstrate their expertise to their organization, the public, the palliative care community, and the health sector.	Achieves specialty palliative certification as a demonstration of ongoing commitment to integrate and apply the knowledge, skills, and judgment with the attitudes, values, and beliefs required to practice safely, effectively, and ethically in a designated role and setting and advocates certification for all specialty palliative nurses. The APRN commits to ongoing certification to ensure quality care in a changing environment.
Advocacy	The association that serves as the leading voice for individuals, families, and nurses to transform the care and culture of serious illness.	Participates in policy development and legislation processes for issues and concerns that pertain to the care of individuals with serious illness and nursing's role in healthcare. They advocate for individuals with serious illness, their families, and other nurses.
Leadership	The association that empowers its nurse members to transform the culture and care of individuals with serious illness with expert palliative nursing.	Leads and influences change within an area of palliative care including, but not limited to: clinical practice, education, research, advocacy, administration, and measurement.
Research and Scholarship	The association that translates evidence about the care and culture of serious illness into action.	Focuses on health outcomes for individuals and families and the nurse's role in those outcomes. They initiate, participate, publish, and contribute to research, as well as disseminate findings.
Clinical practice	The association that facilitates expert clinical practice delivery.	Delivers expert evidence-based palliative nursing, including expert assessment of the physical, psychological, emotional, spiritual, and cultural domains of care; complex pain and symptom management; skilled communication surrounding advance care planning and goals of care; grief and loss support; and navigation of ethical dilemmas.

Palliative and hospice APRNs have a significant role and are essential to palliative care delivery, quality, and access, more than ever before. Nurse practitioners represent the largest growing segment of healthcare professionals. With healthcare reform, palliative and hospice APRNs will drive change by their increased presence and role in relieving work force shortages. These revised competencies reflect the maturity of the specialty of palliative nursing. They are a guide for palliative and hospice APRN role delineation as well as a roadmap for establishing expertise and proficiency expectations as palliative advanced practice nursing matures.

—Constance Dahlin, MSN, ANP-BC, ACHPN, FPCN, FAAN

References

1. American Nurses Association. Recognition of a Nursing Specialty, Approval of a Specialty Nursing Scope of Practice Statement, Acknowledgement of Specialty Nursing Standards of Practice, and Affirmation of Focused Practice Competencies. American Nurses Association; 2017. Accessed January 11, 2021. https://www.nursingworld.org/~4989de/globalassets/practiceandpolicy/scope-of-practice/3sc-booklet-final-2017-08-17.pdf
2. Dahlin C, ed. *Palliative Nursing: Scope and Standards of Practice,* 6th ed; Hospice and Palliative Nurses Association; 2021.
3. Dahlin C, Coyne P. History of the advanced practice role in palliative nursing. In: Dahlin C, Coyne P, Ferrell B, eds. *Advanced Practice Palliative Nursing.* Oxford University Press; 2016: 3-12.
4. Promoting Excellence in End-of-Life Care. *Advanced Practice Nurses Role in Palliative Care - A Position Statement from American Nurse Leaders.* Promoting Excellence; 2002. Accessed January 11, 2021. https://www.promotingexcellence.org/apn/pe3673.html
5. Hospice and Palliative Nurses Association. *HPNA Position Statement: Value of the Advanced Practice Registered Nurse in Palliative Care.* Pittsburgh, PA: Hospice and Palliative Nurses Association, 2015. https://advancingexpertcare.org/position-statements Accessed January 11, 2021.
6. Dahlin C, Coyne P. The palliative APRN leader. *Ann Palliat Med.* 2019. 8(Suppl 1):S30-S38. doi:10.21037/apm.2018.06.03
7. Hospice and Palliative Credentialing Center. Advanced Certified Hospice and Palliative Nurse. Certification Verification Tool. Accessed January 11, 2021. https://advancingexpertcare.org/HPNA/Certification/Credentials/APRN_ACHPN/HPCC/CertificationWeb/ACHPN.aspx?hkey=fe8a39d4-bbe7-4acf-83c2-a13d29670579
8. National Consensus Project for Quality Palliative Care. *Clinical Practice Guidelines for Quality Palliative Care.* 4th ed. National Hospice and Palliative Care Coalition; 2018. Accessed January 11, 2021. https://www.nationalcoalitionhpc.org/ncp/
9. Dahlin C, Moreines Tycon L, Root M, eds. *Core Curriculum for the Hospice and Palliative APRN.* 3rd ed. Hospice and Palliative Nurses Association; 2020.
10. Hospice and Palliative Nurses Association. HPNA Mission, Vision, and Pillars of Excellence. 2020. Accessed January 11, 2021. https://advancingexpertcare.org/HPNA/About/Mission_Strategic_Plan/HPNA/About_Us/About.aspx?hkey=63b4511d-eba6-4c88-b732-4685a5988b6d.
11. Dahlin C. *The Hospice and Palliative APRN Professional Practice Guide.* Hospice and Palliative Nurses Association; 2017.

Palliative and Hospice Advanced Practice Registered Nurse Competencies

The Palliative and Hospice APRN Role

The palliative and hospice advanced practice registered nurse (APRN) has a prominent role in addressing individual, professional, and societal needs associated with the experience of serious illness from diagnosis to death. Palliative care is defined as "patient and family-centered care that optimizes quality of life by anticipating, preventing, and treating suffering. Palliative care throughout the continuum of illness involves addressing physical, intellectual, emotional, social, and spiritual needs and to facilitate patient autonomy, access to information, and choice."[1 p.4]

The focus of palliative care is on individuals with serious illness, including progressive chronic illnesses that adversely affect an individual's daily functioning as well as will predictably reduce life expectancy. Care is provided in a holistic manner that promotes quality of life and optimizes function through symptom management, and psychosocial and spiritual support to myriad populations in a collaborative manner, across the life span from perinates, neonates to older adults, and across diverse health settings.

There are two roles in advanced palliative nursing practice: the palliative advance practice registered nurse (APRN), and the graduate-level prepared palliative and hospice nurse (APN) (See Table 2).[2,3] The role of the palliative and hospice advanced practice registered nurse (APRN) is the focus of these competencies. Palliative and hospice APRNs have completed graduate education at the master's or doctoral level to practice as nurse practitioners (NPs) and clinical nurse specialists (CNSs) and have attained expertise in the subspecialty of palliative care.

Within palliative nursing, the palliative and hospice APRN is distinguished by their ability to synthesize complex data, implement plans of care, and provide leadership in palliative care.[4] Accordingly, the palliative and hospice APRN may function in many roles: expert clinician, leader, educator, researcher, consultant, collaborator, advocate, case manager, administrator, program developer, and policy maker. It is through these many roles that palliative and hospice APRNs promote access to quality care for a wide range of individuals.

The palliative and hospice APRN has fulfilled the requirements established by individual state nurse practice acts. In palliative care, the APRN is usually an NP or a CNS, as these are the roles eligible for specialty certification as an Advanced Certified Hospice and Palliative Nurse (ACHPN). However, the majority of states follow the regulations as delineated by the National Council of State Boards of Nursing, which states that the palliative and hospice APRN must have concurrent advanced practice certification in a primary APRN population foci.[5] Within palliative care, five of the six foci are common for APRN practice: family practice, adult-gerontology, neonatal, pediatrics, and psychiatric-mental health APRNs are working in the community and the acute care setting.[5] This means that certification as an ACHPN is a secondary or specialty certification in addition to one's primary practice.

The second role of advanced practice nurses (APNs) is graduate-level prepared palliative and hospice nurses who are educated at the master's and/or doctoral level such as a PhD, DNS, DNSc, MSN, or MS. Their licensure for clinical practice is at the registered nurse level and their specialty certification is a certified hospice and palliative nurse (CHPN), a certified hospice and palliative pediatric nurse (CHPPN) or a certified hospice and palliative care administrator (CHPCA). They are held to the competencies of the palliative and hospice registered nurse (RN). In addition, there are legal and professional distinctions between an APRN and an RN (regardless of academic achievements) who provides care at a highly expert level due to extensive experience. The nurse who has been working for many years as a registered nurse is a very valuable member of the palliative team. However, the experienced registered nurse cannot be considered an APRN without having graduate-level preparation as an NP, CNS, certified nurse midwife (CNM), or certified registered nurse anesthetist (CRNA), and licensure as an APRN.

Table 2. Two APN Roles[2,3]

Role	Preparation	Licensure	ANA Definition	Hospice and Palliative Nursing Certification
APRN	Clinical Doctorate DNP Master's MSN, MS	APRN	• Completes an accredited graduate-level education program preparing one for the role of certified nurse practitioner, certified registered nurse anesthetist, certified nurse midwife, or clinical nurse specialist • Passes a national certification examination that measures the APRN role and population-focused competencies • License to practice as an APRN • Maintains continued competence as evidenced by recertification	ACHPN
APN	Research Doctorate PhD, DNS, DNSc Master's MS, MA, MSN in education	RN	• A registered nurse educationally prepared and then licensed by a state, commonwealth, territory, or government regulatory body to practice as a registered nurse • Education at the master's or doctoral educational level who has advanced knowledge, skills, abilities, and judgment • Functions in an advanced level as designated by elements of her or his position	CHPN, CHPPN

This knowledge and expertise afford palliative and hospice APRNs a high level of responsibility and scope of practice to deliver palliative care. Within the spectrum of clinical care, APRNs provide symptom management, optimize function, care coordination, advanced care planning, and enhance quality of life. Providing care, APRNs exercise a high degree of critical thinking, analysis, and independent judgment within the framework of autonomous and collaborative interdisciplinary practice. Depending on the state in which an APRN practices, and their role as an NP or a CNS, they may be authorized to assume autonomous responsibility for clinical role functions, which includes assessment and clinical evaluation; diagnosis; management; completion of advance care planning documents in accordance with state practice acts; and prescription of therapies, medications, or controlled substances. The range of clinical settings of the hospice and palliative APRN are represented, such as acute care, rehabilitation, skilled nursing facilities, long-term care settings, home settings, and all hospice settings. In all these settings, and by their advance level of practice, it is significant that the palliative and hospice APRN is eligible for reimbursement for the services they provide.

Overview of Competencies

The use of standards and competencies and the requirements for primary and specialty certification are necessary to delineate practice. As required by ANA, specialty scope and standards describe the nature of a nursing specialty in terms of the work of the professional and the responsibility of the specialty within itself and to the public.[3] As stated in the Foreword, *Palliative Nursing: Scope and Standards of Practice* defines palliative nursing practice to the nursing profession, the palliative nursing community, and the field of palliative care.[3,6] Specifically, it delineates the who, what, where, when, how, and why of palliative nursing—who benefits from palliative nursing, what palliative nursing does, where palliative nursing is delivered, when palliative nursing is delivered, how palliative nursing is delivered, and why palliative nursing is a specialty.[6]

Competencies are the actions that reflect the integration of knowledge, skills, experience, and attitudes to meet the needs of individuals, families, healthcare organizations, and the public. Of note, there are graduate-level competencies for primary palliative nursing that complement these specialty competencies.[7] This document, however, describes the explicit intellectual, interpersonal, technical, and moral competencies necessary for quality advanced practice palliative nursing that are outcome-specific and measurable. By virtue of graduate education and related clinical expertise, it is expected that APRNs demonstrate a greater depth and breadth of knowledge, skills, theory, research, and practice that are reflected in these competencies.[8,9] All APRNs demonstrate these eight competencies. However, each nurse must determine which of the advanced core behaviors within each competency best matches their educational, preparation, practice, and licensure.

The definition of competency has evolved and been adapted over time. In this edition, there are several defining aspects of competency that guide this document. ANA defines a competency as an "expected level of performance that integrates knowledge, skills, abilities, and judgment" and "an expected and measurable level of nursing performance that integrates knowledge, skills, abilities, and judgment, based on established scientific knowledge and expectations for nursing practice."[2,10] As applied to advanced practice palliative nursing, competencies are the quantifiable behaviors necessary to further advanced practice palliative nursing. Thus, the *Competencies for the Palliative and Hospice Advanced Practice Registered Nurse* are the quantifiable knowledge, attitudes, and skills that palliative and hospice APRNs demonstrate in the delivery of safe, evidence-based, high-quality, empathetic, state-of-the-art, serious illness care, while ensuring care is congruent to individuals' and families' beliefs, preferences, and wishes.

The *Competencies for the Palliative and Hospice Advanced Practice Registered Nurse* represent "a greater depth and breadth of knowledge and an ability to synthesize complex data to develop, implement, and coordinate comprehensive holistic individual-centered plans of care with goals of maximizing health, quality of life, and functional capacity."[11 p. 2] In this edition, the competencies were revised to provide synergy with guiding tenets of practice and knowledge expectations for the APRN within foundational documents and the consensus of experts. The initial groundwork of this edition is the work of palliative APRN clinical and academic faculty who educate, train, mentor, and cultivate palliative APRNs, listed as Contributers.[12,13] Foundational documents underpin the competencies including: a) the 2020 Hospice and Palliative Nurses Association's *Palliative Nursing: Scope and Standards of Practice* approved by the American Nurses Association, b) the 2020 Hospice and Palliative Nurses Association's *Core Curriculum for the Hospice and Palliative Advanced Practice Registered Nurse;* c) the 2018 National Consensus Project for Quality Palliative Care's *Clinical Practice Guidelines for Quality Palliative Care;* and d) the 2020 detailed content outline behavioral expectations for certification as outlined by the Hospice and Palliative Credentialing Center (HPCC) for advanced certification in hospice and palliative nursing (ACHPN).[6,9,14,15]

With their broad application to all settings and populations, the Competencies for the Palliative and Hospice Advanced Practice Registered Nurse provide a foundation for the development of educational goals and objectives that determine expectations for skills and knowledge for ideal advanced practice palliative nursing. They can frame specialty content in graduate nursing programs, palliative APRN fellowships, palliative APRN residencies, palliative APRN onboarding, and with various other educational programs. These competencies apply to:

- Palliative and hospice APRNs working with all populations of individuals with serious illness across the life span from perinatal care to geriatric care.
- Care delivered across all settings where individuals receive healthcare: skilled nursing facilities, clinics, residential home settings (e.g., home, group homes, shelters), acute care settings, community settings (e.g., schools, community centers).
- All types of healthcare encounters, whether virtual or in-person.

Building on the core competencies of the palliative registered nurse, advanced practice palliative nursing competencies reflect advanced knowledge, skills, and attitudes that palliative advanced practice nurses obtain through master's, post-master's and doctoral education in both clinical care and nonclinical work. Specifically, the competencies are appropriate for APRNs in providing evidence-based care in the four quality-of-life domains: physical, psychosocial, emotional, and spiritual care to individual and families experiencing serious illness.[6,14]

Palliative and Hospice Advanced Practice Registered Nurse Competency Model

Competencies must be framed in a model of practice. The Hospice and Palliative Nurses Association has long adopted the American Association of Critical Care Nurses (AACN) *Synergy Model for Patient Care* as its framework. The core concept of this model is that "characteristics of patients and families influence and drive the characteristics or competencies of nurses."[16] This is harmonious with the focus of palliative nursing being patient-centered and family-focused for all age groups. Specifically, the following assumptions about individuals and families are essential to palliative nursing practice:[16 p 1-2]

- Individuals are biological, psychological, social, and spiritual entities who present at a particular developmental stage. The whole of the individual (body, mind, and spirit) must be considered.
- The individual, family, and community all contribute to providing a context for the nurse-patient relationship.
- A goal of nursing is to restore an individual to an optimal level of wellness as defined by the individual. Death can be an acceptable outcome, in which the goal of nursing care is to move an individual toward a peaceful death.

Palliative and Hospice Advanced Practice Registered Nursing Roles

The *Synergy Model* outlines eight roles of nursing practice: Clinical Judgement, Advocacy and Moral Agency, Caring Practices, Collaboration, Response to Diversity, Systems Thinking, Facilitation of Learning, and Clinical Inquiry. Each *Synergy Model* role was tailored to reflect the palliative nursing role within the scope and standards.[3,6] The *Palliative Nursing: Scope and Standards of Practice* were written for the registered nurse, with additional statements for advanced practice nurse and advanced practice registered nurse. Therefore, each *Synergy Model* role was refined to reflect the advanced education and scope of practice of the APRN to guide the necessary knowledge, skills, and attitudes within the advanced nursing role. It is assumed that the nursing process is consistent among all populations and it tailored to the age, development, and cognition of the individual with serious illness, and includes their family or caregiver.

Clinical Judgment

Within palliative care, the palliative nurse demonstrates clinical judgment, clinical reasoning, critical thinking, and decision-making surrounding palliative nursing, integrating global knowledge of multidimensional needs of individuals with serious illness and their families using the nursing process.

Advocacy and Moral Agency

The palliative nurse integrates knowledge, attitudes, behaviors, and skills that are consistent with nursing professional standards, nursing codes of ethics, and scope of practice into their palliative nursing practice. This includes advocating for human rights of all individuals, with the goal of addressing and reducing health disparities, inequities, racism, and discrimination against people of color, LGBTQ+ persons, and other marginalized groups.

Caring Practices

The palliative nurse integrates caring practices to create a compassionate, supportive, and therapeutic environment for individuals with serious illness, families, and staff, including vigilance, engagement, and responsiveness.

Collaboration

The palliative nurse collaboratively engages with individuals with serious illness, their families, and healthcare providers, in a way that promotes each person's contributions toward achieving optimal yet realistic individual and family goals.

Systems Thinking

The palliative nurse identifies and utilizes the evidence and body of knowledge for palliative care delivery and clinical practice, as well as the tools to manage the environmental and system resources, for the individual with serious illness, their family, and staff within a healthcare system and a community.

Response to Diversity

The palliative nurse has the cultural sensitivity to recognize, appreciate, and incorporate the cultural needs and preferences of individuals with serious illness into the provision of care. Assessment includes but is not limited to cultural identity, spiritual beliefs, sexual orientation, gender identity, gender expression, ethnic identity, socioeconomic status, age, educational level, and values.

Facilitation of Learning

The palliative nurse facilitates learning for individuals with serious illness, their families, nurse colleagues, other members of the healthcare team, and the community.

Clinical Inquiry

The palliative nurse utilizes the ongoing process of questioning and evaluating palliative practice and providing informed practice based on the established palliative care research evidence and related information.

Competencies are necessary to delineate the knowledge, skills, attitudes, and behaviors of practice to protect the public and the specialty's integrity. The Competencies for the Palliative and Hospice Advanced Practice Registered Nurse are the quantifiable knowledge, attitudes, and skills that palliative and hospice APRNs demonstrate in the performance of serious illness care that is safe, evidence-based, high-quality, empathetic, state-of-the-art, and congruent to individuals' and families' beliefs, preferences, and wishes. They are grounded in a solid foundation of history, and evidence base in alignment with current nursing practice to the ANA Nursing: Scope and Standards, the HPNA Palliative *Nursing: Scope and Standards of Practice*, the NCP *Clinical Practice Guidelines* and the AACN *Synergy Model*.[2,6,14,16]

References

1. U.S. Department of Health and Human Services, Centers for Medicare and Medicaid Services (CMS), Center for Clinical Standards and Quality/Survey and Certification Group. (2012). *CMS Publication 100-07 State Operations, Provider Certification.* September 27, 2012. Accessed January 11, 2021. https://www.cms.gov/Medicare/Provider-Enrollment-and-Certification/SurveyCertificationGenInfo/Downloads/Survey-and-Cert-Letter-12-48.pdf

2. American Nurses Association. *Nursing Scope and Standards of Practice.* 3rd ed. American Nurses Association; 2015.

3. American Nurses Association. *Recognition of a Nursing Specialty, Approval of a Specialty Nursing Scope of Practice Statement, Acknowledgement of Specialty Nursing Standards of Practice, and Affirmation of Focused Practice Competencies.* American Nurses Association; 2017. Accessed January 11, 2021. https://www.nursingworld.org/~4989de/globalassets/practiceandpolicy/scope-of-practice/3sc-booklet-final-2017-08-17.pdf.

4. Centers for Medicare and Medicaid Services, Medicare Learning Network. *Advanced Practice Registered Nurses, Anesthesiologist Assistants, and Physician Assistants.* Vol 2020. Department of Health and Human Services. 2020. Accessed January 11, 2021. https://www.cms.gov/Outreach-and-Education/Medicare-Learning-Network-MLN/MLNProducts/Downloads/Medicare-Information-for-APRNs-AAs-PAs-Booklet-ICN-901623.pdf.

5. APRN Consensus Work Group, National Council of State Boards of Nursing APRN Advisory Committee. *Consensus Model for APRN Regulation: Licensure, Accreditation, Certification, and Education.* National Council of State Boards of Nursing; 2008. Accessed January 11, 2021. https://www.ncsbn.org/aprn-consensus.htm

6. Dahlin C, ed. *Palliative Nursing: Scope and Standards of Practice.* 6th ed. Hospice and Palliative Nurses Association; 2021.

7. American Association of Colleges of Nursing. Primary palliative care competencies for master's and DNP nursing students: (G-CARES) Graduate competencies and recommendations for educating nursing students. American Association of Colleges of Nursing, 2019. Accessed January 11, 2021. https://www.aacnnursing.org/Portals/42/ELNEC/PDF/Graduate-CARES.pdf.

8. Whitehead P, Dahlin C, eds. *Compendium for Non-Cancer Diagnoses.* 3rd ed. Hospice and Palliative Nurses Association.; 2019.

9. Dahlin C, Moreines Tycon L, Root M, eds. *Core Curriculum for the Hospice and Palliative APRN.* 3rd ed. Hospice and Palliative Nurses Association; 2020.

10. American Nurses Association. Position Statement: Professional Role Competence. American Nurses Association; 2014. Accessed January 11, 2021. https://www.nursingworld.org/practice-policy/nursing-excellence/official-position-statements/id/professional-role-competence/.

11. Hospice and Palliative Nurses Association. HPNA Position Statement: Value of the Advanced Practice Registered Nurse in Palliative Care. Hospice and Palliative Nurses Association; 2015. Accessed January 11, 2021. https://advancingexpertcare.org/position-statements

12. Dahlin C, Ersek M, Wholihan D, Wiencek C. Specialty Palliative APRN Practice Through State-of-the-Art Graduate Education: Report of the HPNA Graduate Faculty Council (SA509). Abstract for the Annual Assembly. *J Pain Symptom Manage.* 2019;57(2):445.

13. Dahlin C, Wholihan D, Johnstone-Petty M. Palliative APRN fellowship guidelines—a strategy for quality specialty practice: report of the HPNA APRN Fellowship Council (TH300). Abstract for the Annual Assembly. *J Pain Symptom Manage.* 2019;57(2):383.

14. National Consensus Project for Quality Palliative Care. *Clinical Practice Guidelines for Quality Palliative Care.* 4th ed. National Hospice and Palliative Care Coalition; 2018. Accessed January 11, 2021. https://www.nationalcoalitionhpc.org/ncp/

15. Hospice and Palliative Credentialing Center. Advanced Certified Hospice and Palliative Nurse. 2020. Accessed January 11, 2021. https://advancingexpertcare.org/HPNA/Certification/Credentials/APRN_ACHPN/HPCC/CertificationWeb/ACHPN.aspx

16. American Association of Critical-Care Nurses. *Synergy model for patient care* 2nd ed. American Association of Critical-Care Nurses; 2018. Accessed January 11, 2021. https://www.aacn.org/nursing-excellence/aacn-standards/synergy-model

Palliative and Hospice APRN Competencies

Clinical Judgment

Advanced Practice Palliative Nursing Competency Statement: The palliative and hospice APRN demonstrates advanced clinical judgment, clinical reasoning and decision-making as appropriate to advanced practice nursing, based on expert knowledge and skill in the assessment (history, current concerns and physical examination), diagnosis, planning, and management of complex human responses, and the integration of global knowledge of the multidimensional needs of individuals with serious illness and their families.

Clinical Judgment: Advanced Practice Nursing Core Behaviors
- Conducts an advanced, comprehensive, or problem-focused assessment, in-person, virtually, or via telehealth, of individuals and families experiencing serious illness, including current concerns, physical, functional, emotional, social, cultural, spiritual, and quality-of-life aspects.
- Obtains a health history, including presenting signs and symptoms, course of disease or condition, past and current disease or condition, and directed therapies for cure or palliation from multiple sources of data.
- Determines the individual's and their family's or caregiver's understanding of health status and illness.
- Determines the goals, values, preferences, and concerns of individuals with serious illness, their families, as well as health colleagues in order to promote shared, informed decision-making.
- Performs an advanced physical examination to determine relevant physical findings.
- Orders and interprets common screening and diagnostic tests in context of the goals of care for the individual with serious illness.
- Assesses risk factors for substance use disorder, stratifies and mitigates risk, and practices universal precautions for opioid use for all individuals.
- Orders, analyzes, and interprets assessment and diagnostic data to make accurate clinical and differential diagnoses for pain and other symptoms, including but not limited to dyspnea, nausea, vomiting, constipation, diarrhea, anxiety, depression, delirium, fatigue, and anorexia for individuals with serious illnesses.
- Prioritizes health problems of individuals and families experiencing serious illness based on collaboratively derived interdisciplinary goals of care.
- Identifies a disease trajectory and outcomes based on advanced critical analysis of both complex assessment data and relevant diagnoses, expert knowledge of pathophysiology and disease progression, and with consideration of the benefits and burdens of care.
- Assesses and manages psychological distress and psychiatric syndromes based on evidence-based practice.
- Prescribes, recommends, and implements palliative interventions informed by evidence-based practice to alleviate physical, psychological, emotional, social, and spiritual symptoms associated with serious illness, which may include pharmacotherapeutics, nonpharmacological interventions, complementary and integrative therapies in accordance with an individual's preferences and resources.
- Evaluates and revises the unique plan of care for individuals with serious illness and their families based on their evolving needs and preferences and the complex, competing, and shifting priorities in goals of care.

- Deviates from the standard of care or applies knowledge from other realms when necessary to prevent, reduce, or resolve suffering in the individual living with serious illness.
- Identifies individual and family needs for resources and obtains consent for appropriate referrals for additional care, services, and support, including hospice, within a palliative care context.
- Provides strategies and resources to support individuals with serious illness and families experiencing loss, grief, and bereavement, including coping strategies via in-person visits or through technology.
- Plans for site of death, attendance of family or community members, and other treatments or procedures as commensurate with individual's and family's values, wishes, and desired rituals.
- Documents an accurate, comprehensive, and problem-focused palliative care assessment and plan of care for individuals and their families with serious illness, recording the extent of provided services, and appropriate coding to communicate complexity of services delivered within a palliative care consultation note, evaluation note, or follow-up note.
- Assumes responsibility for one's own overall evaluation, documentation, and communication of palliative care assessment and plan of care to enhance the continuity and quality of palliative care across healthcare settings.
- Coordinates the execution of a comprehensive holistic care, including pain and symptom management, psychological, emotional, social, and spiritual support reflecting the diversity of the individual and their family.
- Synthesizes and utilizes evidence-based palliative care outcome data to inform and improve quality of care delivery within the healthcare delivery system.
- Applies relevant information and communication technologies, conceptual models, theories, and research in developing, implementing, and evaluating comprehensive, evidence-based, effective, efficient, and compassionate palliative care.

Advocacy and Moral Agency

Advanced Practice Palliative Nursing Competency Statement: The palliative and hospice APRN integrates knowledge, attitudes, behaviors, and skills that are consistent with, and assume responsibility of, advanced practice nursing professional standards, nursing codes of ethics, and advanced practice scope of practice within their care delivery. The palliative and hospice APRN serves as a moral agent to identify and resolve moral and ethical concerns, including advocating for human rights of all individuals, with the goal of addressing and reducing health disparities, inequities, racism, and discrimination.

Advocacy and Moral Agency: Advanced Practice Nursing Core Behaviors

- Practices in accordance with the professional standards of the American Nurses Association's (ANA) *Nursing: Scope and Standards of Practice* and HPNA's *Palliative Nursing: Scope and Standards of Practice a*s well as the *ANA Code of Ethics for Nurses* and *HPNA's Code of Ethical Conduct which* articulate the moral foundation of palliative and hospice advanced practice nursing.[1-4]
- Assumes accountability of advanced palliative nursing practice with the incorporation of all appropriate federal laws, regulations, and standards from *Centers for Medicare and Medicaid Services (CMS) for APRNs,* state statutes, regulations and laws as well as currently accepted professional standards of advanced practice nursing into own's practice.[5]
- Maintains expected certification and licensure requirements for advanced practice palliative nursing in accordance with institutional, state, and federal laws and regulations, as well as specialty and professional nursing organizations' certification requirements.
- Articulates and practices within the legal limits of palliative care and the role of the APRN in accordance with state advance nursing practice statutes and organizational bylaws, including disclosure of health information and medical records; medical decision-making by the APRN; advance care planning and directives and the APRN; the roles and responsibilities of surrogate decision-makers; APRN controlled substance prescription; APRN death pronouncement and certification processes; autopsy requests; organ and anatomical donation; and healthcare documentation expectations by the APRN.
- Evaluates one's own practice, the practice of one's APRN colleagues, and one's interdisciplinary colleagues in palliative and hospice care with regard to institutional, state, and federal laws and regulations.
- Articulates the significance of advanced practice palliative nursing and uses opportunities to promotes the role of the hospice and palliative APRN in palliative care and healthcare systems.
- Role models ethical conduct in advance palliative nursing practice, seeking input from colleagues, ethics committees, and legal counsel.
- Assesses the individual with serious illness with attention to populations at risk (e.g., older adults; children and youths; persons experiencing homelessness; persons of color; LGBTQ+ persons; persons experiencing substance abuse disorders; persons with serious mental illness; individuals without legal validation; individuals incarcerated in jails, prisons, and detention centers; persons with cognitive impairment, as well as developmental, intellectual, and physical disabilities) in an age, cognitive, and developmentally appropriate manner.
- Articulates disparities in care associated with cultural differences, spiritual beliefs, sexual orientation, gender identity, gender expression, race, ethnicity, socioeconomic status, and age.
- Articulates the impact of health disparities, social injustices, discrimination, racism, oppression, and trauma on individuals, families, and communities, particularly as it pertains to delivery of palliative care and how to mitigate them.
- Collaborates with the palliative interdisciplinary team, other health team professionals, and the public to protect human rights, promote health diplomacy, enhance cultural sensitivity and congruence, and reduce health disparities.

- Collaborates with other health professionals to ensure ethically sound organizational systems for access to and fair distribution of healthcare resources across all populations.
- Communicates at the advanced level to facilitate informed decision-making including treatment options, risks, burdens, benefits, and outcomes of healthcare regimens through informed consent, informed assent, and refusal or decline of treatments and therapies.
- Assesses an individual's capacity for decision-making, and identifies appropriate surrogate decision-maker(s) and seek consultation for legal determination of competency consistent with policies and statutes.
- Adheres to legal and regulatory requirements for disclosure, decision-making capacity assessment, confidentiality, and informed consent, as well as informed assent and permission for individuals who are not of legal age to consent.
- Acknowledges and promotes age and developmentally appropriate discussions concerning care of individuals with serious illness.
- Adheres to the rights of children in decision-making with respect to developmental stage and cognitive capacity, as appropriate to population foci of practice.
- Incorporates the principles of "'best interest'" versus "'harm'" to help establish the threshold where a parental decision can be overridden in the care of children or a surrogate decision-maker in adults who lack decision-making capacity, in collaborating with ethics and legal representatives in complex situations.
- Incorporates advanced facilitation skills through open discussion of divergent views and develop a plan for continued communication.
- Reviews the health record for an individual's expressed wishes documentation of advance care planning documents, documents them in health care record, revises and updates them as appropriate and advocates for them across settings of care through the plan of care.
- Completes advance care planning and documents with the individual with serious illness that reflect the individual's wishes (e.g., designation of surrogate decision-maker, advanced directives, living wills, signing of hospital orders for life sustaining treatment order sets such as provider/physicians/medical orders for life-sustaining treatments [POLST/ MOLST] as per state regulations).
- Maintains confidentiality while communicating data, plans, and results in a manner that preserves the privacy and dignity of the individual and family for all manners of care, including care delivered via in-person, virtual and telehealth.
- Describes what health information is mandated to be shared, why it must be shared, and with whom it will be shared with individuals with serious illness and families.
- Uses appropriate terminology, format, and technology to convey care plan and advance care planning documents to other appropriate health providers.
- Uses a systematic approach to ethical and legal review of clinical and palliative-related healthcare issues in collaboration with an ethics committee and legal counsel, particularly in the development of palliative-related policies and procedures, incorporating ethical principles (i.e., beneficence, autonomy, justice, non-maleficence, veracity), and consulting ethics resources/services as appropriate.
- Articulates and provides ethical care in customary palliative care situations including but not limited to decision-making capacity, surrogate decision-making, an individual's right to decline treatments of any kind; use of high-dose medications; discontinuation of life sustaining therapies (e.g., antibiotics, pressors, ventilators, dialysis, ventricular assist devices, antibiotics); palliative sedation; the appropriateness of complex treatments or non-beneficial medical treatments; cessation of oral nutrition and medically administered nutrition and hydration, requests for medically administered death, and the use of cannabis and psychedelics.

- Assesses, develops, implements, and evaluates organizational structures to support quality palliative care, such as policies and procedures for quality improvement and research projects, ethics consultation, and legal counsel.
- Develops, implements, and evaluates strategies to overcome individual clinician, and healthcare system obstacles, as well as social, legal, or economic barriers to palliative care, pain and symptom management, and healthcare delivery.
- Leads and supports the team and organization in situations of conflict with public health guidelines in palliative care situations or in times of local, regional, or national health crises and humanitarian crises caused by natural disasters (e.g., earthquakes, fire, floods, hurricanes, tsunamis, volcano eruptions), mass casualties, conflict (e.g., war, political and ethnic strife), epidemics and public health crises (e.g., pandemics—infections; epidemics—opioids, systematic racial injustice), and nuclear accidents, when it is necessary to change focus from person-centered practice supported by clinical ethics to clinical care guided by public health ethics.[6,7]

Caring Practices

Advanced Practice Palliative Nursing Competency Statement: The palliative and hospice APRN integrates advanced caring practices to create a compassionate, supportive, and therapeutic environment for individuals with serious illness (perinates, neonates, children, adolescents, young adults, and older adults) and their families with the aim of promoting comfort, healing and preventing unnecessary suffering. This is accomplished by, but is not limited to, vigilance, engagement, and responsiveness to themselves, individuals, families, and other healthcare providers.

Caring Practices: Advanced Practice Nursing Core Behaviors
- Maintains personal self-identity while mindfully acknowledging the similarities and differences between self and the individual with serious illness's values and goals.
- Demonstrates compassion and respect for the inherent dignity, worth, and unique attributes of all people.
- Cultivates an open, flexible approach with individuals and families, focusing on their needs and differentiating them from the needs of the healthcare team and one's personal needs.
- Promotes physical, psychological, social, emotional, and spiritual care of self and other palliative care colleagues.
- Monitors and considers one's own emotional response to interaction with individuals and families experiencing serious illness using self-reflective practice.
- Integrates caring practices, including self-kindness, empathy, equanimity, authentic presence, respect, allowance of time, and caring consciousness for self-care, development, and professional transcendence within advanced palliative nursing practice.
- Identifies symptoms of personal emotional distress, moral injury, moral distress, compassion fatigue, moral residue, burnout, for oneself as well as such symptoms for one's interprofessional team and addresses these symptoms with available resources.
- Develops a personal plan to support well-being, resiliency and sustainability within advanced practice nursing and palliative care.
- Identifies, integrates and advocates for system level resources for clinician well-being.
- Uses effective communication methods, including verbal, nonverbal, and/or symbolic means appropriate to the individual, with particular attention to individuals with cognitive impairment, and appropriate to the developmental stage and cognitive capacity of children, as relevant to one's practice population foci.
- Creates a climate of trust, respect, and partnership between individuals and families with serious illness and interdisciplinary team members in the provision of specialty palliative care.
- Offers therapeutic presence, including silence, with individuals and families experiencing serious illness by providing comfort, emotional support, opportunities for disclosure, and sharing at deeper levels.
- Establishes caring relationships with individuals and families to facilitate coping with sensitive issues.
- Creates an environment of effective and compassionate communication for individuals receiving palliative care, families, healthcare professionals, and community.
- Builds trusting collaborative relationships with staff, APRN colleagues, team members, other disciplines, ancillary services, and the community.
- Uses advanced communication skills to assess and respond to subtle and unique individual and family/caregiver needs, communication styles, strengths, diversity, and safety concerns; developing the ability to anticipate future changes and needs of individuals with serious illness and their families.
- Uses advanced caring behaviors to engage with individual, family and caregivers with patience, respect, emotional intelligence, cultural intelligence, and a caring consciousness.

- Demonstrates effective communication skills that assist individuals and families in identifying their goals and values to inform complex medical decisions.
- Communicates scientific and evidence-based knowledge from electronic and information technologies as required by Centers for Medicare and Medicaid Services (CMS) to individuals and their families to assist with decision-making.
- Facilitates communication, negotiation, and conflict resolution, including the ability to analyze, manage, and negotiate conflict between individuals, families, team members, and other healthcare professionals.
- Promotes interprofessional team respect using opportunities to impart knowledge about APRNs, APRN scope of practice and APRN contribution to care delivery.
- Encourages and supports others to effect change in the healthcare system, based on the application of theory, recognition of mutual respect, and delineated role responsibilities, as well as facilitating the communication of palliative care recommendations.
- Provides appropriate patient-centered health information, instruction, and counseling, using evidence-based rationales for individuals experiencing serious illness and their families regarding decision-making, symptom management, and goals of care and other palliative issues.

Collaboration

Advanced Practice Palliative Nursing Competency Statement: The palliative and hospice APRN collaboratively engages with individuals with serious illness, their families, and healthcare providers, in the provision of palliative care, with the focus on patient-centered and family-focused care, in a way that promotes each person's contributions toward achieving optimal, yet realistic individual and family goals.

Collaboration: Advanced Practice Nursing Core Behaviors
- Builds trusting and collaborative relationships with interdisciplinary team members, health colleagues of all disciplines, healthcare staff, and the community.
- Creates and engages in a formal process to seek feedback regarding one's own palliative practice from individuals, peers, the palliative interdisciplinary team, professional colleagues, and others as well as palliative policies, procedures, and outcomes.
- Develops, implements, and evaluates strategies to effectively collaborate with members of the specialty palliative care team through team-building and recognizing each member's unique role, area of expertise, skills, and contributions.
- Leads an interdisciplinary team approach in the provision of individual-centered and family-focused palliative care through assessment, planning, implementation, and evaluation as defined by the NCP *Clinical Practice Guidelines*.[8]
- Consults with other disciplines and specialty palliative care team members to maximize utilization of palliative nursing skills as related to health education, health promotion, health restoration, and/or health maintenance.
- Collaborates with specialty palliative care team members and other colleagues involved in the individual's care to identify values, preferences, and beliefs that form the basis of the plan of care.
- Collaborates with specialty palliative care team members regarding continuity of care within transitions of care.
- Collaborates with community agencies to facilitate care in the setting preferred by the individual and family, when feasible, including both hospice and home care services provided in a variety of settings.
- Assumes leadership to promote palliative care concepts into the public regarding potential or actual physical, psychological, emotional, social, and spiritual components of living with a serious illness.
- Assumes leadership roles within the specialty palliative care team to execute comprehensive holistic care within the physical, psychological, social, emotional, spiritual, and cultural domains of care.
- Assumes leadership roles in organizing, implementing, and evaluating initiatives to improve the effective delivery of comprehensive palliative care.
- Demonstrates leadership in the roles of clinician, educator, researcher, advocate, mentor, consultant, collaborator, administrator, coordinator, and case manager.
- Collaborates with health professionals and family caregivers across transitions of care including community service agencies, long term care facilities, acute care facilities, hospice, and home health agencies to facilitate seamless transitions of care and care in the setting preferred by the individual and their family.
- Develops collaborative and synergistic relationships with referring providers, consultant providers, and other health care providers by eliciting the perspectives and advice of others regarding patient care, treatment plans, and practice issues.
- Collaborates with specialty palliative care team members and other healthcare professionals to promote consistent communication in patient and family meetings; discussions regarding goals of care, delivery of bad news; and conversations about prognosis and imminent death.

- Develops synergistic relationships with referring providers, consultant providers, and other healthcare providers by eliciting the advice and perspectives of others regarding patient care and practice issues.
- Develops processes for the management of conflict surrounding patient care and work toward consensus building about treatment plans and goals of care.
- Mentors APRN and other palliative colleagues in the acquisition of clinical knowledge, skills, abilities, and management of individuals with serious illness.
- Facilitates active involvement and contributions of others in team activities (e.g., patient care meetings, team support meetings, business meetings, journal club, quality improvement meetings).

Systems Thinking

Advanced Practice Palliative Nursing Competency Statement: The palliative and hospice APRN identifies and utilizes the evidence and body of knowledge for palliative care delivery and advanced clinical practice, as well as the tools to proactively manage the environmental and system resources, for the individual with serious illness, their family, and staff within a health organization, a care system, and a community.

Systems Thinking: Advanced Practice Nursing Core Behaviors

- Demonstrates effectiveness as a team member in various healthcare delivery settings, systems and interprofessional teams relevant to clinical specialty.
- Anticipates needs and advocates for individuals with serious illness and families as they move through the healthcare system.
- Identifies and advocates for the most appropriate setting for the delivery of palliative care for an individual with serious illness and the family consistent with their goals and preferences as they move through the healthcare system.
- Applies relevant information and communication technologies, conceptual models, theories, and research in developing, implementing, and evaluating comprehensive, evidence-based, effective, efficient, and compassionate palliative care.
- Develops, integrates, and applies a variety of advanced treatment interventions driven by needs, strengths, and resources of the individual with serious illness and their family.
- Provides cost-effective, quality palliative care by using the most appropriate resources and delegating appropriate care to qualified nursing colleagues, such as nursing assistants, licensed vocational/practical nurses, and other personnel.
- Considers access, barriers, cost, efficacy, and quality when making palliative care decisions (treatment decisions, prescriptions, referrals) to ensure efficient use of resources for individuals with serious illness.
- Leads the implementation of a global outlook of care delivery across the healthcare system with an understanding of coordinating, negotiating and navigating a system, utilizing untapped and alternate resources as necessary to achieve safe, cost-effective, efficient, timely, person-centered, and equitable care to optimize outcomes for individuals with serious illness.
- Identifies, develops, implements, and evaluates programs and initiatives for integrated palliative care and quality improvement across healthcare settings to promote continuity of care, quality, effectiveness and value.
- Demonstrates stewardship of financial and other resources for the delivery of quality care that is effective, affordable and sustainable; and evaluates quality and cost-effectiveness, including budget, for practice initiatives.
- Articulates the importance of population health principles and apply them to palliative care.
- Maintains current knowledge of healthcare financing, the healthcare organization, financing of the healthcare system, and current trends within healthcare as it affects the delivery of palliative care.
- Utilizes systematic methods to assess the palliative care needs of healthcare systems, healthcare organizations, individuals, and families.
- Utilizes business and management strategies to provide quality palliative care and the efficient use of resources.
- Negotiates and navigates palliative care services and resources for individual with serious illness with appropriate agencies through case management with attention to the most appropriate nursing resources (nursing assistants, licensed vocational/practical nurses, and registered nurses) and other palliative resources from disciplines such as rehabilitation, social work, chaplaincy,

volunteers, pharmacy, and medicine as well as untapped and alternative resources (e.g., expressive therapies, child-life services, and bereavement services).

- Collaborates in the development, implementation, and evaluation of systems level strategies to reduce errors and optimize safe, effective healthcare delivery and reduce barriers to quality palliative care.

- Leads and participates in shaping contemporary healthcare policy at community, local, state, regional, and national levels to improves healthcare outcomes and optimize access to and delivery of safe, quality, cost-effective, healthcare.

- Analyzes systems-level policies considering issues of access, quality and cost, and health disparities through the development and implementation of policies.

- Participates in legislative and policy-making activities that influence, support, and enhance the role and practice of the palliative and hospice advanced practice nurse.

- Evaluates implications and synthesizes information about the impact of contemporary health policy on healthcare providers, individuals and families, and the community who experience serious illness.

- Evaluates health information resources, such as the internet, in the area of practice for applicability, accuracy, readability, and comprehensibility to help individuals with serious illness and their families access quality health information.

- Participates in resource allocation and utilization of primary and specialty palliative care strategies in periods of health and humanitarian crises caused by natural disasters (e.g., earthquakes, fire, floods, hurricanes, tsunamis, volcano eruptions), mass casualties, conflict (e.g., war, political and ethnic strife), public health crises (e.g., pandemics—infections, epidemics—opioids, systematic racial injustice), and nuclear accidents.

- Develops strategies of palliative care programs and systems to meet the needs of its communities, patient populations, and care locations, with particular attention to health, racial, and social disparities.

- Analyzes the impact of caring for individuals with serious illness on family, community, and healthcare systems, including identification of available resources and potential barriers across all healthcare settings.

Response to Diversity

Advanced Practice Palliative Nursing Competency Statement: The palliative APRN has the cultural sensitivity to recognize, appreciate, and incorporate the differing cultural needs of individuals with serious illness into the provision of care, which may include, but not limited to, cultural differences, spiritual beliefs, sexual orientation, gender identity, gender expression, race, ethnicity, lifestyle, socioeconomic status, age, and values.

Response to Diversity: Advanced Practice Nursing Core Behaviors
- Practices in accordance with the HPNA Palliative Nursing: Scope and Standards of Practice; the ANA Code of Ethics for Nurses, the ANA Position Statement The Nurse's Role in Ethics and Human Rights: Protecting and Promoting Individual Worth, Dignity, and Human Rights in Practice Settings, the HPNA Code of Ethical Conduct; and the NCP Clinical Practice Guidelines: Domain 5—Spiritual, Religious, and Existential Aspects of Care and Domain 6—Cultural Aspects of Care.[2,3,8,9]
- Recognizes personal values and biases in the form of self-assessment.
- Maintains appropriate boundaries between individuals' and families' beliefs and values and one's own beliefs and values when delivering quality palliative care.
- Practices with cultural awareness, sensitivity, and humility by performing self-examination of cultural beliefs and values and how they relate to healthcare and the environment in which one works.
- Uses skills, tools, resources, and communication that are appropriately vetted for the culture, literacy, and language of the population served, with emphasis on respect for appropriateness within the themes of palliative care.
- Integrates age and developmentally appropriate aspects of care into the delivery of palliative care acknowledging the different needs of individuals based on the needs of perinates, neonates, children, adolescents, young adults, and older adults, and their families or caregivers.
- Demonstrates cultural intelligence, sensitivity, and humility including spiritual, religious, and existential principles across healthcare settings, which promote health, respect, and assist in managing serious illness experienced by individuals and families.
- Identifies and responds to health disparities, social injustices and racism within palliative care and leads initiatives to mitigate them.
- Demonstrates ability to collect relevant cultural data related to the individual and family presenting health condition and unmet needs; accurately performs culturally specific assessment to deliver culturally competent interdisciplinary palliative care.
- Promotes respect for the individual and family's cultural perceptions, preferences, and practices regarding illness, disability, treatment, help seeking, disclosure, decision-making, grief, death, dying, and family composition.
- Assesses, identifies, and addresses cultural, spiritual, and existential beliefs, behaviors, practices, needs, and concerns of individuals with serious illness and family members according to established protocols and documents in the interdisciplinary care plan.
- Leads person-centered and family-focused care that is respectful of relevant data from a cultural and social assessment pertaining to the individual and family with serious illness, including but not limited to spiritual beliefs, religion, ethnicity, race, sexual orientation, gender identity, gender expression, and socioeconomic status with attention to marginalized populations, such as older adults; children and youths; persons experiencing homelessness; persons of color; LGBTQ+ persons; persons experiencing substance use disorders; persons with serious mental illness; individuals without legal validation; individuals incarcerated in jails, prisons, and detention centers; persons with cognitive impairment, as well as developmental, intellectual, and physical disabilities.

- Accesses appropriate cultural, spiritual, and religious resources to deliver palliative care to individuals and families.
- Explores life review, assessment of hopes, values, and fears; meaning; purpose; beliefs about afterlife; spiritual or religious practices; cultural norms; and beliefs that influence understanding of illness, coping, guilt, forgiveness, life-closure and life-completion tasks.
- Offers support for issues of life closure, as well as other spiritual issues, in a manner consistent with the individual's and the family's cultural, spiritual, and religious values.
- Participates in cross-cultural interactions with individuals' and families' and interdisciplinary teams from culturally diverse backgrounds.
- Recognizes and educates others about diverse systems of belief and the role of diversity in the application of professional health provider obligations, including information on diagnosis; disclosure; decisional authority; care; and acceptance of decisions to continue, discontinue, or forgo treatments.
- Provides culturally and spiritually competent care by incorporating cultural, spiritual, and existential beliefs, behaviors, customs, practices, and ceremonies of individuals and family members into a comprehensive care plan.
- Recognizes and integrates the variances in physiological and psychological responses within cultural, spiritual, religious, racial, ethnic, age, and gender groups that may influence the development of palliative plans of care for individuals with serious illness and their families.
- Addresses conflicts that may arise between individuals, families, and healthcare providers resulting from differences in cultural and spiritual perspectives related to palliative care, and plans for effective strategies to allow for and accommodate those differences.
- Creates and sustains a work environment that affirms diversity, multiculturalism, and respect.

Facilitation of Learning

Advanced Practice Palliative Nursing Competency Statement: The palliative and hospice APRN provides and facilitates learning for individuals with serious illness, their families, nurse colleagues, other members of the healthcare team, and the community in formats appropriate to the environment (i.e., virtual, in-person, or hybrid models).

Facilitation of Learning: Advanced Practice Nursing Core Behaviors
- Self-evaluates practice for areas of strength and areas for further development; modifies advanced palliative nursing practice in response to self-evaluation and peer review.
- Obtains necessary education and/or assistance to meet learning/performance goals and improve one's palliative care advanced nursing practice.
- Demonstrates knowledge, skills, confidence, and competence in the application of learning principles appropriate the individual's developmental and learning needs (i.e., children, adults, and differing abilities) when providing palliative care education to individuals, families, healthcare professionals, and the community inherent in the role of the hospice and palliative APRN.
- Assesses for individual, family, and caregiver level of knowledge, preferred mode of learning, and identifies cues indicative of low levels of health literacy or numeracy.
- Identifies and uses opportunities to facilitate advanced learning about palliative care among individuals, families and caregivers, health colleagues and the public.
- Educates individuals, families, and caregivers with respect to culture, literacy, age, and development.
- Leads palliative care-related communication and teaching-learning experiences framed by respect, humility, time, and a caring consciousness.
- Uses educational methods to support informed decision-making that are consistent with individual, family, and caregiver's preferred mode of learning, literacy, and readiness.
- Foster individual and family understanding of expected course of serious or advanced illness, potential changes in condition, benefit and burdens of potential treatment options, and role of palliative care.
- Evaluates the effectiveness of education and communication strategies using methods, such as the teach back method, with individuals with serious illness and their families.
- Applies principles of literacy and health literacy to promote understanding of disease process, pain and symptom management, end-stage illness, and signs of imminent death.
- Integrates education regarding safe practice and prescribing for pain management, including risk assessment; safe and appropriate storage, use, and disposal; universal precautions in the use of opioids and as appropriate; medication assisted therapy (MAT); prescribing and integration during serious illness; for individuals on palliative care and hospice.
- Integrates education regarding palliative care inequities utilizing contextual data related to health disparities and racial inequities in formal and informal programs.
- Integrates current healthcare research findings and other evidence to expand clinical knowledge, skills, abilities, judgment, and management of individuals with serious illness.
- Creates, provides, and supports educational programs in serious illness care to increase knowledge of professional topics for nurses and other health professionals to enhance role performance.
- Serves as a role model, preceptor, mentor, and facilitator of learning in advanced palliative nursing practice to enhance skills in both primary and specialty APRN practice.
- Analyzes the impact of social, political, and economic influences and human health exposures on the global palliative care environment and takes appropriate action to advocate for the field of palliative care and individuals living with serious illness.

- Refers individuals and families to evidence-based resources, including additional information and guidance about serious illnesses, treatment options, advance care planning, and support agencies.
- Educates caregivers regarding expected course of serious illness, potential changes in conditions, along with the benefit and burdens of potential treatment options to support informed decision-making in management of serious illness with respect to culture, literacy, age, and development.
- Provides information to individuals, families, and caregivers concerning medications, intended effects, adverse effects, safekeeping, and disposal.
- Develops, implements, and evaluates formal and informal education in palliative care for individuals, families, healthcare professionals, and the community.
- Provides education that influences individual, professional, and societal attitudes regarding palliative care.
- Disseminates current, evidence-based palliative care education to health professionals and the general population at the local, state, regional, and national levels.
- Promotes palliative care education through graduate palliative nursing practicums and preceptorships, APRN palliative fellowships and residencies and continuing education.
- Contributes to professional development and education directed toward improving individual, family, community, and environmental outcomes and improving their professional growth.
- Participates actively in professional and specialty nursing organizations related to advanced palliative nursing practice and care of individuals with serious illness.
- Publishes research, education, and clinical findings in professional journals in areas of care of individuals with serious illness.
- Shares knowledge through presentations at professional meetings to contribute to hospice and palliative care, and the palliative and hospice advanced practice nursing role.
- Contributes to the identification of future education and research, as well as to the development of creative and innovative ways for advanced palliative nursing practice to improve care delivery and outcomes.

Clinical Inquiry

Advanced Practice Palliative Nursing Competency Statement: The palliative and hospice APRN continually questions and evaluates advanced palliative nursing practice and palliative care and provides informed practice based on the established palliative care research evidence and related information. In addition, the palliative and hospice APRN uses research to promote improved outcomes for individuals with serious illness and the community.

Clinical Inquiry: Advanced Practice Nursing Core Behaviors
- Integrates quality palliative nursing in clinical practice, education, administration, and research.
- Leads care delivery towards palliative outcomes that reflect an individual's healthcare culture, values, and ethical concerns.
- Evaluates the efficacy and optimal ordering of diagnostic tests, clinical procedures, therapies, and treatment plans to optimize quality of life function and reduce suffering in partnership with the individual with serious illness and their family.
- Leads, designs, organizes and evaluates quality-improvement studies, research initiatives, and programs to improve palliative outcomes and care of individuals with serious illness in diverse settings.
- Creates palliative metrics and measures (structure, process, or outcome measures) that incorporate clinical effectiveness, patient satisfaction, continuity, consistency, and expenditures among providers.
- Utilizes research to identify, examine, validate, and evaluate current theories and palliative care practice, with the goal of improved outcomes for individuals with serious illness, their families, and the community.
- Engages in the ongoing process of questioning, developing, implementing, and evaluating advanced practice palliative nursing through policies, procedures, and guidelines.
- Creates and directs practice changes in palliative care through research utilization and experiential learning.
- Individualizes and applies validated pain and symptom assessment tools, treatment protocols, practice standards, and palliative practice guidelines to inform diagnosis, treatment, and evaluation of individuals with serious illness.
- Utilizes information technology, (i.e., research information and databases), to locate the current, best available evidence and guidelines to support palliative care interventions and advanced practice palliative nursing.
- Advances, leads and participates in the ongoing improvement of the quality and safety of palliative care practice through team-based and organization-based quality improvement interventions and research activities.
- Designs quality-improvement studies, research initiatives, and programs to improve palliative outcomes and care of individuals with serious illness in diverse settings.
- Promotes advanced practice palliative nursing through scholarly inquiry, professional development, and the generation of policy.
- Applies knowledge obtained from advanced educational preparation in nursing or other related areas, as well as current research and evidence, to clinical decision-making at the point of care to achieve optimal palliative care outcomes.
- Uses available benchmarks as a means to evaluate palliative nursing practice at the individual, departmental, and organizational levels.
- Demonstrates ability to critically examine and review research related to serious illness care to identify, validate, evaluate, and improve palliative care practice and outcomes.
- Serves as a liaison to institutional, local, state, regional, and national legislative bodies to influence issues relating to care in advanced palliative nursing practice, with the goal of improved

outcomes for the individual, family, institution, community, and environment related to the potential or actual disease process and treatments.

- Develops practice standards, protocols, policies, and other documents based on synthesis of evidence-based literature that address clinical issues, quality improvement, and expected palliative related outcomes.
- Evaluates individual, family, community, and environmental outcomes related to health, wellness, illness processes, and treatments.
- Utilizes current research and evidence-based findings and participates in ongoing educational activities to expand advanced clinical knowledge and to enhance performance of the advanced palliative registered nurse.
- Initiates inquiry into comprehensive databases in order to utilize available research related to palliative care and to support evidence-based practice.
- Evaluates the quality of research, clinical articles, internet, or web-based information related to palliative care.
- Utilizes information systems for the storage and retrieval of data related to individuals and families experiencing serious illness.
- Participates in and supports palliative research that validates best practices in the care of individuals and families dealing with serious illness.
- Applies scientific methods to analyze outcomes, validate quality, impact change, and improve palliative care practice.

Definitions

Advanced Practice Registered Nurse. A registered nurse who has completed an accredited graduate-level education program preparing her or him for the role of certified nurse practitioner, certified registered nurse anesthetist, certified nurse-midwife, or clinical nurse specialist; has passed a national certification examination that measures the APRN role and population-focused competencies; maintains continued competence as evidenced by recertification; and is licensed to practice as an APRN.[1 p. 85]

Caring. The moral ideal of nursing consisting of human-to-human attempts to protect, enhance, and preserve humanity and human dignity, integrity, and wholeness by assisting a person to find meaning in illness, suffering, pain, and existence.[10]

Code of ethics (nursing). A list of provisions that makes explicit the primary goals, values, and obligations of the nursing profession and expresses its values, duties, and commitments to the society of which it is a part. In the United States, nurses abide by and adhere to *Code of Ethics for Nurses with Interpretive Statements*.[3]

Collaboration. A professional healthcare partnership grounded in a reciprocal and respectful recognition and acceptance of: each partner's unique expertise, power, and sphere of influence and responsibilities; the commonality of goals; the mutual safeguarding of the legitimate interest of each party; and the advantages of such a relationship.[1 p. 85]

Competency. An expected and measurable level of nursing performance that integrates knowledge, skills, abilities, and judgment, based on established scientific knowledge and expectations for nursing practice.[1 p. 85]

Environment. The surrounding habitat, context, milieu, conditions, and atmosphere in which all living systems participate, and interact. It includes the physical habitat as well as the cultural, psychological, social, and historical influences. It includes both the external space as well as an individual's internal physical, mental, emotional, social and spiritual experiences.[1]

Evaluation. The process of determining the progress toward the attainment of expected outcomes, including the effectiveness of care.[1]

Evidence-based practice. A scholarly and systematic problem-solving paradigm that results in the delivery of quality healthcare. Evidence-based practice is the conscientious use of current best evidence in making decisions about patient care.[11] It is a problem-solving approach to clinical practice and administrative issues that integrates a systematic search for and critical appraisal of the most relevant evidence to answer a burning clinical question, one's own clinical expertise, or patient preferences and values.[12]

Expected outcomes. End results that are measurable, desirable, and observable, and translate into observable behaviors.[1]

Graduate-level prepared registered nurse. A registered nurse prepared at the master's or doctoral educational level who has advanced knowledge, skills, abilities, and judgment; functions in an advanced level as designated by elements of her or his position; and is not required to have additional regulatory oversight.[1 p. 87]

Illness. The subjective experience of discomfort, disharmony, or imbalance.

Individual with serious illness. The person with a diagnosis of a serious or advanced illness who is the central focus of palliative care. This person is the one to whom the registered nurse provides services, as sanctioned by state regulatory bodies. The individual with serious illness may be an infant, child, adolescent, young adult, adult, or older adult who has a chronic illness and is dependent on others; has various disabilities; has advanced illness; or has a terminal illness.

Interdisciplinary team. An interdisciplinary team (IDT) provides services to the individual and family consistent with the care plan. In addition to chaplains, nurses, physicians, and social workers, other therapeutic disciplines who provide palliative care services to individuals and families may include: child-life specialists; nursing assistants; nutritionists; occupational therapists; respiratory therapists; pharmacists; physical therapists; massage, art, and music therapists; psychologists; and speech and language pathologists.[13] Integrates separate discipline approaches into a single consultation. That is, the patient history taking, assessment, diagnosis, intervention, and short- and long-term management goals are conducted by the team, together with the individual, and at one time rather than separately addressing the individual.[14]

Interprofessional. Reliant on the overlapping knowledge, skills, and abilities of each professional team member. This can drive synergistic effects by which outcomes are enhanced and become more comprehensive than a simple aggregation of the individual efforts of the team members. Interprofessional education occurs when two or more professions learn about, from, and with each other to enable effective collaboration and improve health outcomes.[13,15]

Registered nurse. Individual who is educationally prepared and then licensed by a state, commonwealth, territory, or government regulatory body to practice as a registered nurse. "Nurse" and "professional nurse" are synonyms for a registered nurse in this document.

Scope of nursing practice. Description of the "who," "what," "where," "when," "why," and "how" of nursing practice for all registered nurses. Each question must be answered to provide a complete picture of the dynamic and complex practice of nursing and its evolving boundaries and membership. The scope of practice in conjunction with the *Nursing Scope and Standards* and the *Code of Ethics for Nurses with Interpretive Statements* comprehensively describe the competent level of nursing common to all registered nurses.[1,3]

Serious or life-limiting illnesses. A health condition that carries a high risk of mortality and either negatively impacts a person's daily function and/or quality of life or excessively strains the caregiver.[8,16] It can also include conditions and treatments in which the conditions pose significant burden. These occur in all populations of individuals of all ages (perinates, neonates, children, adolescents, and adults).

Social determinants of health (nonmedical factors influencing health). Aspects of human health, including quality of life, which are determined by physical, chemical, biological, social, political, and psychological conditions in the environment in which people are born, grow, work, live, and age. It refers to the theory and practice of assessing, correcting, controlling, and preventing those factors in the environment that can potentially adversely affect the health of present and future generations.[17]

Specialty palliative nursing. Includes the management of individuals with serious, advanced illness or trauma injury with complex and refractory symptoms, advanced skills in communication and conflict resolution, and navigating the changing care needs across the trajectory of life. Specialty palliative nursing is provided by both registered nurses and advanced practice registered nurses. Specialty palliative care occurs in a variety of settings and across disease populations (e.g., oncology, heart failure, pediatrics, geriatrics, pulmonology).[8,13]

Standards of practice. Statements that describe a competent level of nursing care demonstrated by the critical thinking model known as the nursing process. The nursing process encompasses significant actions taken by registered nurses and forms the foundation of the nurse's decision-making.[1]

Standards of professional nursing practice. Authoritative statements of the duties that all registered nurses, regardless of role, population, specialty, setting, or APRN foci, are expected to competently perform. These published standards may serve as evidence of the standard of practice and care, with the understanding that application of the standards depends on context.[1]

Standards of professional performance. Statements that describe a competent level of behavior in the professional role. All registered nurses are expected to engage in professional role activities reflective of their education, experience, and position.[1]

References

1. American Nurses Association. *Nursing Scope and Standards of Practice.* 3rd ed. American Nurses Association; 2015.
2. Dahlin C, ed. *Palliative Nursing: Scope and Standards of Practice.* 6th ed. Hospice and Palliative Nurses Association; 2021.
3. American Nurses Association. *Code of Ethics for Nurses with Interpretive Statements.* American Nurses Association; 2015.
4. Hospice and Palliative Nurses Association. Code of Ethical Conduct. Accessed January 11, 2021. https://advancingexpertcare.org/ethical-conduct
5. Centers for Medicare and Medicaid Services, Medicare Learning Network. Advanced Practice Registered Nurses, Anesthesiologist Assistants, and Physician Assistants. Vol 2020. Department of Health and Human Services; 2020. Accessed January 11, 2021. https://www.cms.gov/Outreach-and-Education/Medicare-Learning-Network-MLN/MLNProducts/Downloads/Medicare-Information-for-APRNs-AAs-PAs-Booklet-ICN-901623.pdf
6. Berlinger N, Wynia M, Powel T. Ethical Framework for Health Care Institutions Responding to Novel Coronavirus SARS-CoV-2 (COVID-19). *Guidelines for Institutional Ethics Services Responding to COVID-19. Managing Uncertainty, Safeguarding Communities, Guiding Practice.* The Hastings Center; 2020. Accessed January 11, 2021. https://www.thehastingscenter.org/ethicalframeworkcovid19/
7. World Health Organization. *Integrating Palliative Care and Symptom Relief into the Response to Humanitarian Emergencies and Crises: A WHO guide.* World Health Organization; 2018. Accessed January 11, 2021. https://www.who.int/publications-detail/integrating-palliative-care-and-symptom-relief-into-the-response-to-humanitarian-emergencies-and-crises
8. National Consensus Project for Quality Palliative Care. *Clinical Practice Guidelines for Quality Palliative Care.* 4th ed. National Hospice and Palliative Care Coalition; 2018. Accessed January 11, 2021. https://www.nationalcoalitionhpc.org/ncp/
9. American Nurses Association. *Position Statement: The Nurse's Role in Ethics and Human Rights: Protecting and Promoting Individual Worth, Dignity, and Human Rights in Practice Settings.* American Nurses Association; 2016. Accessed January 11, 2021. https://www.nursingworld.org/~4af078/globalassets/docs/ana/ethics/ethics-and-human-rights-protecting-and-promoting-final-formatted-20161130.pdf
10. Watson J. Caring Science and Human Caring Theory. 2020. Accessed January 11, 2021. https://www.watsoncaringscience.org/jean-bio/caring-science-theory/
11. Straus S, Glasziou P, Richardson S, Haynes R. *Evidence based medicine: How to practice and teach EBM.* 5th ed. Elsevier; 2019.
12. Melnyk B, Fineout-Overholt E. *Evidence-Based Practice in Nursing & Healthcare: A Guide to Best Practice.* 4th ed. Walters Kluwer; 2019.
13. American Nurses Association, Hospice and Palliative Nurse Association. A Call for Action - Nurses Lead and Transform Palliative Care. American Nurses Association, 2017. Accessed January 11, 2021. http://www.nursingworld.org/CallforAction-NursesLeadTransformPalliativeCare
14. Davis K. Understanding the importance of the interdisciplinary team in pediatric hospice. National Hospice and Palliative Care Organization; 2018. Accessed January 11, 2021. https://www.nhpco.org/wp-content/uploads/2019/04/PALLIATIVECARE_UnderstandingIDT.pdf.
15. World Health Organization. Health Professions Networks, Nursing and Midwifery, Human Resources for Health. Framework for Action on Interprofessional Education & Collaborative Practice. World Health Organization; 2010. Accessed January 11, 2021. https://www.who.int/hrh/resources/framework_action/en/
16. Kelley A, Bollens-Lund E. Identifying the populations with serious illness: the "denominator" challenge. *J Palliat Med.* 2018;21(S2):S7-S16.

17. World Health Organization. Social Determinants of Health Unit. Department of Public Health, *Environmental and Social Determinants of Health.* World Health Organization, 2017. Accessed January 11, 2021. https://www.who.int/social_determinants/SDH-Brochure-May2017.pdf?ua=1